Contents

INTRODUCTION

Attempts to quantify glucose in the urine date back to the mid-1800s and laid the foundation for modern diabetes care. The most important development in the commercialization of urine glucose testing came in 1908, when Benedict developed a copper reagent for urine glucose, which was used, with some modifications, for more than 50 years (1). The cumbersome methodology of heating became more convenient in 1945 with the development of Clinitest (Ames, Elkhart, IN), which featured a modified copper reagent tablet. Glucose was oxidized, and the amount of glycosuria was proportional to the color of the heated solution.

In 1965, Ames developed the first blood glucose test strip, the Dextrostix, using glucose oxidase. A large drop of blood was placed on the strip and, after 60 seconds, was washed away. The generated color was then compared to a chart on the bottle for a semi-quantitative assessment of blood glucose. This early strip was for physicians' offices, not for home use.

The first glucose meter was used in the 1970s with the Dextrostix, but its precision and accuracy were poor. By the mid-1970s, the concept of patients using blood glucose data at home was contemplated, and by 1980, the Dextrometer was launched; this meter used the Dextrostix along with a digital display. During the 1980s, meters and strips requiring less blood became available, all at a cheaper price. Self-monitoring of blood glucose (SMBG) became the standard of care, especially for patients with type 1 diabetes. This advance, along with A1C testing and insulin pump therapy, made possible the Diabetes Control and Complications Trial, which positively answered the long debate about the relationship between glucose control and diabetes complications.

Through the late 1980s, 1990s, and early 2000s, SMBG technology continued to improve. The blood removal step was eliminated, smaller amounts of blood were required, electrochemical strips were developed, wider ranges of hematocrit were permitted, and new enzymatic tests were used. Lancets also improved. By 2010, SMBG was virtually painless and recommended for all patients receiving insulin and most who were not.

The evolution of home glucose monitoring was further revolutionized with the introduction of continuous glucose monitoring (CGM). In 1999, the U.S. Food and Drug Administration approved the first "professional" CGM, with which the patient was blinded to glucose data collected for 3 days, and then the information was downloaded in the health care provider's office for review.

Until recently, all CGM devices required calibration with fingerstick blood glucose measurements. The first "real-time" CGM was the Glucowatch Biographer (Cygnus, Redwood, CA).

This device was worn as a wristwatch using "reverse iontophoresis" to stimulate the secretion of subcutaneous fluid, from which glucose was measured using an electrode. The Glucowatch was not a commercial success, owing in large part to site irritation despite the fact that the sensor was technically noninvasive.

In 2004, Medtronic (Northridge, CA) introduced the Guardian REAL-Time CGM system, which could notify users of potentially dangerous hyperglycemia or hypoglycemia, and by 2006, the same company released the first integrated pump and sensor. That same year, Dexcom (San Diego, CA) introduced its first real-time CGM, called the STS (Short-Term Sensor). In 2008, the FreeStyle Navigator by Abbott (Alameda, CA) was released in the United States. All of the initial CGM devices required blood glucose confirmation for insulin decisions to be made.

Dexcom introduced the G4 Platinum in 2012. In 2015, the G5 Mobile was launched, now allowing data to be transmitted to a user's cell phone (similar to the G6, which was launched in 2018). Medtronic also had improvements in technology, with the next-generation professional CGM, the iPro, released in 2008. Medtronic's second-generation integrated pump-sensor device became available in 2009, and in 2013, the loop came closer to being closed with the introduction of the MiniMed 530G Enlite sensor, the first pump with "threshold suspend" for hypoglycemia. Medtronic's first hybrid closed-loop device was available in 2017 using the Guardian Sensor 3. Over time, the accuracy of all of these sensors improved.

Abbott introduced the FreeStyle Libre Pro in 2016. This professional CGM is the first that requires no fingerstick testing during wear. It also is unique in that the sensor can be worn for 14 days. As with earlier professional CGM systems, data are blinded to the user until they are downloaded and reviewed with the health care provider. The FreeStyle Libre, for direct use by patients, became available in the United States in late 2017 but earlier in other countries. In the United States, it has a 12-hour warm-up time and can be worn for 10 days. Like the Pro, it is factory-calibrated; unlike Dexcom or Medtronic CGM devices, it does not sound alarms for out-ofrange glucose levels. The system includes a reader that patients can swipe or "flash" to obtain a glucose reading and trend data (or communicates with a phone in some countries).

In less than 20 years, CGM has revolutionized the way diabetes is managed, especially type 1 diabetes. Evidence supporting the use of CGM is now vast and unequivocal. In this compendium, we review the critical aspects of CGM to assist providers in their daily practice.

Glucose is a 6-carbon structure with the chemical formula C6H12O6. Carbohydrates are ubiquitous energy sources for every organism worldwide and are essential to fuel aerobic and anaerobic cellular respiration in simple and complex molecular forms. Glucose often enters the body in isometric forms such as galactose and fructose (monosaccharides), lactose and sucrose (disaccharides), or starch (polysaccharides). Excess glucose is stored in the body as glycogen, a glucose polymer, utilized during fasting. In addition, glucose can be produced through gluconeogenesis, a process involving the breakdown of fats and proteins. Given the paramount importance of carbohydrates in maintaining homeostasis, numerous sources contribute to glucose production.

The sugar molecule travels through the blood to energy-requiring tissues when glucose is in the body. Glucose undergoes a series of biochemical reactions, releasing energy as adenosine triphosphate (ATP). ATP derived from these processes fuels virtually every energy-requiring process in the body. In eukaryotes, most energy derives from aerobic (oxygen-requiring) processes, which start with a glucose molecule. Glucose is initially broken down through the anaerobic process of glycolysis, producing some ATP and pyruvate as end products. Under anaerobic conditions, pyruvate converts to lactate through reduction. Conversely, under aerobic conditions, the pyruvate can enter the citric acid cycle to generate energy-rich electron carriers that produce ATP at the electron transport chain.

Cellular Level

Glucose reserves are stored as the polymer glycogen in humans. Glycogen is present in the highest concentrations in the liver and muscle tissues. The regulation of glycogen, and thus glucose, is primarily controlled by the peptide hormones insulin and glucagon. These hormones are produced in the pancreatic islet of Langerhans—glucagon from α-cells and insulin from β-cells. The balance between these 2 hormones depends on the body's metabolic state, whether fasting or energy-rich, with insulin in higher concentrations during energy-rich states and glucagon during fasting. Through signaling cascades regulated by these hormones, glycogen is either catabolized, liberating glucose promoted by glucagon during fasting, or synthesized, further consuming excess glucose facilitated by insulin during times of energy abundance. Insulin and glucagon, among other hormones, also control glucose transport in and out of cells by altering the expression of glucose transporter type 4 (GLUT-4).

Several glucose transporters are in the human body, with differential expression varying by tissue type. These transporters are differentiated into 2 main categories—sodium-dependent transporters (SGLTs) and sodium-independent transporters (GLUT).

The SGLTs rely on the active transport of sodium across the cell membrane, which then diffuses down the concentration gradient along with a glucose molecule, known as secondary active transport. The sodium-independent transporters do not rely on sodium and transport glucose using facilitated diffusion. Of the sodium-independent transporters, only GLUT4's expression is affected by insulin and glucagon. The most important classes of glucose transporters and their characteristics are listed below (see Image. Glucose Transporters).

SGLT: Found primarily in the renal tubules and intestinal epithelia, SGLTs are essential for glucose reabsorption and absorption. This transporter works through secondary active transport as it requires ATP to actively pump sodium out of the cell and into the interstitial space through sodium/potassium exchange to establish a favorable concentration gradient for the SGLT. The SGLT between the renal tubule lumen and the intracellular space uses the passive transport of sodium into the cell to drive the cotransport of glucose into the cell.

GLUT-1: Found primarily in the pancreatic β-cells, red blood cells, and hepatocytes. This bi-directional transporter is essential for glucose sensing by the pancreas, an important aspect of the feedback mechanism in controlling blood glucose with endogenous insulin.

GLUT-2: Found primarily in hepatocytes, pancreatic β-cells, intestinal epithelium, and renal tubular cells. This bi-directional transporter is essential for regulating glucose metabolism in the liver.

GLUT-3: This transporter is found primarily in the central nervous system and has a high affinity for glucose, consistent with the brain's increased metabolic demands.

GLUT-4: Found primarily in skeletal muscle, cardiac muscle, adipose tissue, and brain tissue. This transporter gets stored in cytoplasmic vesicles in an inactive state, which merges with the cell membrane when stimulated by insulin. These transporters undergo a 10- to 20-fold increase in density during times of energy abundance upon insulin release with the net effect of a decrease in blood glucose. Glucose more readily enters the cells that have GLUT-4 on their surface.

The end products of carbohydrate digestion in the alimentary tract are predominantly glucose, fructose, and galactose, with glucose comprising 80% of the end product. After absorption from the alimentary canal, a significant portion of the fructose and almost all of the galactose rapidly convert into glucose in the liver. Therefore, only a small quantity of fructose and galactose is present in the blood. Thus, glucose is the final common pathway for transporting all carbohydrates to the tissue cells.

In liver cells, appropriate enzymes are available to promote interconversions among the monosaccharides glucose, fructose, and galactose. The dynamics of the enzymes are such that when the liver releases the monosaccharides, the final product is always glucose. The reason is that the hepatocytes contain a large amount of glucose phosphatase. Glucose-6-phosphate can be broken down into glucose and phosphate, and glucose is transported through the liver cell membrane and back into the blood.

Organ Systems Involved

Glucose is essential for the proper functioning of every organ system. However, specific organs are particularly crucial in regulating its levels.

Liver

The liver plays a crucial role in regulating blood glucose levels. Glycogen, a multibranched polysaccharide of glucose, is the storage form of glucose in the human body, primarily found in the liver and skeletal muscle. Glycogen functions as the body's short-term storage of glucose, whereas triglycerides in adipose tissues serve as the long-term storage. Glucose is released from glycogen when stimulated by glucagon and during fasting conditions, thereby increasing blood glucose levels. Glucose is added to glycogen under the control of insulin and energy-rich conditions, lowering blood glucose levels.

Pancreas

The pancreas releases the hormones that are primarily responsible for controlling blood glucose levels. When glucose concentration rises within the β-cells, Insulin is released, leading to a decrease in blood glucose through various mechanisms outlined below.

Conversely, when glucose levels drop and insulin levels decrease (directly influenced by low glucose levels), α-cells of the pancreas release glucagon, which raises blood glucose through several mechanisms. In addition, somatostatin is released from γ-cells of the pancreas and has a net effect of decreasing blood glucose levels.

Adrenal Gland

The adrenal gland consists of the cortex and the medulla, which play roles in glucose homeostasis. The adrenal cortex releases glucocorticoids, notably cortisol, which raise blood glucose levels through the mechanisms described below. The adrenal medulla releases epinephrine, increasing blood glucose levels through the following mechanisms.

Thyroid Gland

The thyroid gland is responsible for the production and release of thyroxine. Thyroxine affects nearly all tissues in the body, including raising blood glucose levels.

Anterior Pituitary Gland

The anterior pituitary gland releases adrenocorticotropic and growth hormones, increasing blood glucose levels.

Hormones

Many hormones are involved in glucose homeostasis. Understanding each hormone's mechanism and net effect is essential. Remembering which ones lower glucose levels, primarily insulin and somatostatin, can help understand their functions. The other hormones increase glucose levels.

Insulin: Decreases blood glucose levels through increased expression of GLUT4, increased expression of glycogen synthase, inactivation of phosphorylase kinase (thus decreasing gluconeogenesis), and decreased expression of rate-limiting enzymes involved in gluconeogenesis.

Glucagon: Increases blood glucose levels through increased glycogenolysis and gluconeogenesis.

Somatostatin: Decreases blood glucose levels through local suppression of glucagon release and suppression of gastrin and pituitary tropic hormones. This hormone also decreases insulin release; however, the net effect is decreased blood glucose levels.

Cortisol: Increases blood glucose levels through the stimulation of gluconeogenesis and the antagonism of insulin.

Epinephrine: Increases blood glucose levels through glycogenolysis (glucose release from glycogen) and increased fatty acid release from adipose tissues, which can be catabolized and enter gluconeogenesis.

Thyroxine: Increases blood glucose levels through glycogenolysis and increased absorption in the intestine.

Growth hormone: Promotes gluconeogenesis, inhibits liver uptake of glucose, stimulates thyroid hormone, and inhibits insulin.

Adrenocorticotropic hormone: Stimulates cortisol release from adrenal glands and promotes the release of fatty acids from adipose tissue, contributing to gluconeogenesis.

Fasting Blood Glucose Test

This test is standard to measure glucose levels in the bloodstream after an overnight fast of at least 8 hours. The sample is typically collected before breakfast to ensure fasting conditions. Blood glucose levels are assessed using enzymatic assays or automated laboratory analyzers to determine glucose concentration in the plasma or serum. Normal fasting blood glucose levels typically range from 70 to 100 mg/dL (3.9 to 5.6 mmol/L).

Random Blood Glucose Testing

This test is a valuable diagnostic tool for assessing blood glucose levels without fasting or preplanning. The sample is analyzed using a glucometer or laboratory assay to determine the glucose concentration in the bloodstream. Unlike fasting glucose tests or oral glucose tolerance tests, the test provides an immediate snapshot of blood glucose levels, facilitating rapid clinical decision-making. In patients without diabetes mellitus, normal glucose levels typically range from 70 to 140 mg/dL (3.9 to 7.8 mmol/L).These values may vary slightly depending on the laboratory reference range and patient-specific factors.

Oral Glucose Tolerance Test

This test is valuable in assessing glucose metabolism, offering insights into the body's response to ingested glucose. The test aids in the early detection of diabetes and pre-diabetes mellitus, enabling timely interventions to prevent or delay disease progression and associated complications. The test involves administering a standardized oral glucose load, typically 75 g, after an overnight fast, followed by serial blood glucose measurements at specified intervals, typically 0, 30, 60, 90, and 120 minutes post-glucose ingestion. Blood samples are collected to assess glucose concentrations, reflecting the body's ability to handle a glucose challenge.

Normal response: In individuals with normal glucose tolerance, blood glucose levels rise temporarily following glucose ingestion but return to fasting levels within 2 hours. Normal oral glucose tolerance test results indicate efficient glucose uptake and insulin secretion, indicative of intact glucose metabolism.

Impaired glucose tolerance: Impaired glucose tolerance is characterized by elevated blood glucose levels during the oral glucose tolerance test, exceeding normal thresholds but not meeting the diagnostic criteria for diabetes mellitus. This condition represents an intermediate stage of dysglycemia, placing individuals at risk of developing diabetes mellitus and cardiovascular complications.

Diabetes mellitus is diagnosed when the oral glucose tolerance test reveals sustained hyperglycemia, with fasting glucose ≥126 mg/dL (7.0 mmol/L) or 2-hour post-load glucose levels ≥200 mg/dL (11.1 mmol/L) on 2 separate occasions. The oral glucose tolerance test is particularly useful for diagnosing gestational diabetes mellitus, a transient form of diabetes mellitus occurring during pregnancy.

Glucose metabolism is intricately regulated to meet cell energy demands while preventing hyperglycemia or hypoglycemia. The dysregulation of glucose homeostasis underlies the pathogenesis of several metabolic disorders, posing significant health challenges worldwide. Understanding the pathophysiology of glucose dysregulation provides insights into the molecular mechanisms driving metabolic disorders.

Type 1 diabetes: Type 1 diabetes results from autoimmune destruction of pancreatic β-cells, leading to insulin deficiency. Insulin secretion loss impairs peripheral tissue glucose uptake, resulting in hyperglycemia and metabolic derangements.

Type 2 diabetes: Type 2 diabetes primarily arises from insulin resistance, characterized by diminished cellular response to insulin. Peripheral tissues fail to efficiently utilize glucose, leading to compensatory hyperinsulinemia, β-cell exhaustion, and eventual pancreatic dysfunction.

Reactive hypoglycemia: Reactive hypoglycemia occurs postprandially due to excessive insulin secretion in response to carbohydrate-rich meals. This exaggerated insulin release leads to rapid glucose clearance, resulting in hypoglycemic episodes.

Fasting hypoglycemia: Fasting hypoglycemia can stem from various etiologies, including hormonal deficiencies, liver disease, or metabolic enzyme deficiencies, disrupting the balance between glucose production and utilization during fasting periods.

Metabolic syndrome: Metabolic syndrome encompasses a cluster of metabolic abnormalities, including central obesity, insulin resistance, dyslipidemia, and hypertension, predisposing individuals to cardiovascular disease and type 2 diabetes. Insulin resistance plays a central role in the pathogenesis of metabolic syndrome, driving aberrant glucose and lipid metabolism.

Clinical Significance

The pathology associated with glucose often occurs when blood glucose levels are too high or too low. The following summarizes some of the more common pathological states linked to alterations in glucose levels and the associated pathophysiology.

Hyperglycemia

Hyperglycemia can induce pathology, both acutely and chronically. Type 1 and 2 diabetes are both disease states characterized by chronically elevated blood glucose levels that, over time and with poor glucose control, lead to significant morbidity. Both types of diabetes have multifocal etiologies—type 1 is associated with genetic, environmental, and immunological factors and most often presents in pediatric patients, whereas type 2 is associated with comorbid conditions such as obesity in addition to genetic factors and is more likely to manifest in adulthood.

Type 1 diabetes results from the autoimmune destruction of pancreatic β-cells and insulin deficiency, whereas type 2 diabetes results from peripheral insulin resistance due to metabolic dysfunction, often in the setting of obesity. In both cases, the result is inappropriately elevated blood glucose levels, which can lead to pathology through various mechanisms.

- **Osmotic damage:** Glucose is osmotically active and can cause damage to peripheral nerves.
- **Oxidative stress:** Glucose participates in several reactions that produce oxidative byproducts.
- **Non-enzymatic glycation:** Glucose can form complexes with lysine residues on proteins, leading to structural and functional disruption.

These mechanisms lead to various clinical manifestations through both microvascular and macrovascular complications. Some include peripheral neuropathies, poor wound healing or chronic wounds, retinopathy, coronary artery disease, cerebral vascular disease, and chronic kidney disease. Understanding the mechanisms behind the pathology caused by elevated glucose levels is imperative.

High blood sugar levels can also lead to acute pathology, most often observed in patients with type 2 diabetes, known as a hyperosmolar hyperglycemic state. This state occurs when severely elevated blood glucose levels increase plasma osmolality. The high osmolarity leads to osmotic diuresis (excessive urination) and dehydration. A variety of clinical manifestations emerge, including altered mental status, motor abnormalities, focal and global central nervous system dysfunction, nausea, vomiting, abdominal pain, and orthostatic hypotension.

Hypoglycemia

Hypoglycemia is most commonly observed iatrogenically in patients with diabetes mellitus secondary to glucose-lowering drugs. This condition occurs, especially in the inpatient setting, with the interruption of the patient's usual diet. The symptoms are non-specific, but clinical findings such as relation to fasting or exercise and symptom improvement with glucose administration make hypoglycemia more likely.

Hypoglycemia symptoms can be described as either neuroglycopenic, due to a direct effect on the central nervous system, or neurogenic, due to sympatho-adrenergic involvement. Neurogenic symptoms can be further broken down into either cholinergic or adrenergic. The following are some common symptoms of hypoglycemia.

- **Neuroglycopenic:** Fatigue, behavioral changes, seizures, coma, and death.
- **Neurogenic:** Adrenergic such as anxiety, tremor, and palpitations.
- **Neurogenic:** Cholinergic such as paresthesias, diaphoresis, and hunger.

Taking into account what we have learned about glucose in a brief overview of glucose metabolism, let us consider the sequence of events following a carbohydrate-dense meal. Various glucose polymers are broken down in saliva and intestines, releasing free glucose. This glucose is absorbed into the intestinal epithelium through SGLT receptors apically and then enters the bloodstream through GLUT receptors on the basolateral wall. The blood glucose levels spike, triggering an increased glucose concentration in the pancreas and prompting the release of pre-formed insulin. Insulin has several downstream effects, including increased expression of enzymes involved in glycogen synthesis, such as glycogen synthase in the liver. The glucose enters hepatocytes and is added to glycogen chains. Insulin also stimulates the release of GLUT-4 from their intracellular confinement, increasing basal glucose uptake into muscle and adipose tissue as blood glucose levels dwindle. Insulin levels decrease to the low-normal range. As the insulin levels drop below the normal range, glucagon from pancreatic α-cells is released, promoting a rise in blood glucose levels through glycogenolysis and gluconeogenesis. Typically, this increases glucose levels enough to last until the next meal. However, if the patient continues to fast, the adrenomedullary system secretes cortisol and epinephrine, establishing euglycemia from a hypoglycemic state.

Hyperglycemia Symptoms, Causes, and Treatments

What is hyperglycemia

Hyperglycemia is a condition in which the level of glucose in the blood is higher than normal. Sometimes called "high blood sugar," it commonly affects people who have diabetes mellitus, but it can also develop in non-diabetics.

Glucose is the primary source of energy for all cells in our bodies. It comes from the foods we eat, especially carbohydrates. When food reaches the stomach, it is broken down into different parts—one of which is glucose. The intestines absorb the glucose, which then enters the bloodstream and circulates around the body.

Normally, the body uses a hormone called insulin to move glucose from the blood into cells, thereby lowering glucose in the blood and providing cells with energy.

Hyperglycemia can occur when the body does not produce enough insulin or does not respond to insulin correctly. In both cases, glucose stays in the blood instead of being sent to the cells, and as a result, blood glucose levels remain elevated. If more glucose enters the bloodstream—if you eat carbohydrate-rich food, for example—the blood glucose levels climb even higher.

In some cases, people with diabetes who have hyperglycemia can develop a complication called diabetic ketoacidosis (DKA). In this condition, the cells cannot access glucose. Instead, the body gets energy by breaking down fats. This process produces compounds called ketones, which build up in the blood, causing it to become acidic. DKA is a life-threatening condition. (DKA is most commonly associated with type 1 diabetes, but can occur in people with type 2 as well.)

In people with type 2 diabetes, very high blood glucose levels can lead to a life-threatening condition called hyperosmolar hyperglycemic state (HHS), which causes profound dehydration and a change in mental status.

Causes Hyperglycemia

Hyperglycemia most commonly affects people who have diabetes. In type 1 diabetes, the body does not make enough insulin. In type 2 diabetes, the body makes an adequate amount of insulin, but the cells do not respond to it properly. This is called insulin resistance.

For people with diabetes, hyperglycemia can be triggered by:

- Eating too many carbohydrates
- Not exercising enough
- Not taking enough insulin medication (for type 1 diabetes) or other medications that regulate blood glucose levels

Hyperglycemia can also be caused by:

- Medications such as corticosteroids, thiazide diuretics, beta-blockers, and antipsychotics
- Certain conditions that affect the pancreas, which produces insulin
- Medical conditions that can cause insulin resistance, such as Cushing's syndrome and acromegaly

- Pregnancy
- Stress

Risk factors for hyperglycemia

Certain factors or conditions increase the risk for hyperglycemia, including:

- Obesity or being overweight
- Family history of type 2 diabetes
- Personal history of gestational diabetes
- Prediabetes (when blood glucose levels are high, but not high enough to be diagnosed as diabetes)

What are the symptoms of hyperglycemia

Symptoms of hyperglycemia include:

-
- Urinating large amounts
- Excessive thirst
- Feeling tired
- Frequent hunger
- Dry mouth
- Weight loss
- Blurred vision
- Recurrent infections (e.g., urinary infections, skin infections)
- Wounds (cuts, scrapes) that heal slowly

In addition to the symptoms of hyperglycemia, people with DKA may also experience:

- Deep, rapid breathing
- Fruity-smelling breath
- Headache
- Nausea and vomiting
- Stomach pain
- Change in mental status

- Loss of consciousness, coma

HHS can cause the following symptoms:

- Dehydration
- Change in mental status
- Loss of consciousness, coma

Hyperglycemia diagnosis

A diagnosis of hyperglycemia usually involves a review of your medical history, a physical exam, and blood tests.

The doctor will ask about your symptoms and whether you have a family history of diabetes or other risk factors associated with hyperglycemia. He or she will conduct a physical exam.

Ultimately, though, blood tests that measure blood glucose levels are necessary to definitively diagnose hyperglycemia. For what's called a "fasting blood glucose" (FBG) test, you will need to abstain from eating for 8 hours prior to the test. Other blood tests may include a hemoglobin A1C test (also known as glycated hemoglobin test) and an oral glucose tolerance test (OGTT).

Hyperglycemia treatment

The treatment depends on the cause of hyperglycemia, and may include the following:

- Insulin. For people with type 1 diabetes, insulin is the main treatment for hyperglycemia. In some cases, it may also be used to treat people with type 2 diabetes.
- Glucose-lowering medications. Various drugs such as metformin may be used to lower blood glucose levels.
- Glucose monitoring. People with diabetes should monitor their blood glucose levels as instructed by their doctor.
- Lifestyle changes. People with diabetes can reduce the risk of developing hyperglycemia or treat existing hyperglycemia by getting regular exercise, following a nutritious diet, and maintaining a healthy weight.

- DKA and HHS are medical emergencies. They are treated with intravenous fluids, electrolytes, and insulin.

Outlook for people who have hyperglycemia

In general, hyperglycemia that is transient does not cause long-term problems. But if hyperglycemia persists, it can lead to serious complications, including eye problems, kidney damage, nerve damage, and cardiovascular disease.

But with appropriate treatment and regular monitoring of blood glucose levels, people can reduce the risk of hyperglycemia, lower their chances of having serious complications, and live healthy lives.

Yale Medicine unique in its treatment of hyperglycemia

The Yale Diabetes Center provides individualized care for adults with hyperglycemia whether it is transient (such as medication-induced), prediabetes, or type 1 or type 2 diabetes," says Beatrice Lupsa, MD, a Yale Medicine endocrinologist who specializes in type 1 and type 2 diabetes. "Our staff includes endocrinologists, mid-level practitioners, and a dietitian. Our multidisciplinary approach ensures people with blood glucose problems get self-management skills and knowledge to achieve and maintain long-term optimal blood glucose control. We focus on lifestyle interventions, including healthy diet and exercise. Our patients have access to the most advanced medical care, including the latest medications and technologies to prevent hyperglycemic complications and maintain better health throughout their lives.

Hyperglycemia in diabetes

Diagnosis

Your health care provider sets your target blood sugar range. For many people who have diabetes, Mayo Clinic generally recommends the following target blood sugar levels before meals:

Between 80 and 120 milligrams per deciliter (mg/dL) (4.4 and 6.7 millimoles per liter (mmol/L)) for people age 59 and younger who have no medical conditions other than diabetes

Between 100 and 140 milligrams per deciliter (mg/dL) (5.6 and 7.8 millimoles per liter (mmol/L)) for:

People age 60 and older

Those who have other medical conditions, such as heart, lung or kidney disease

People who have a history of low blood sugar (hypoglycemia) or who have difficulty recognizing the symptoms of hypoglycemia

For many people who have diabetes, the American Diabetes Association generally recommends the following target blood sugar levels:

Between 80 and 130 mg/dL (4.4 and 7.2 mmol/L) before meals

Less than 180 mg/dL (10 mmol/L) two hours after meals

Your target blood sugar range may differ, especially if you're pregnant or you have other health problems that are caused by diabetes. Your target blood sugar range may change as you get older. Sometimes, reaching your target blood sugar range can be a challenge.

Home blood sugar monitoring

Routine blood sugar monitoring with a blood glucose meter is the best way to be sure that your treatment plan is keeping your blood sugar within your target range. Check your blood sugar as often as your health care provider recommends.

If you have any symptoms of severe hyperglycemia — even if they seem minor — check your blood sugar level right away.

If your blood sugar level is 240 mg/dL (13.3 mmol/L) or above, use an over-the-counter urine ketones test kit. If the urine test is positive, your body may have started making the changes that can lead to diabetic ketoacidosis. Talk to your health care provider about how to lower your blood sugar level safely.

Hemoglobin A1C test

During an appointment, your health care provider may conduct an A1C test. This blood test shows your average blood sugar level for the past 2 to 3 months. It works by measuring the percentage of blood sugar attached to the oxygen-carrying protein in red blood cells, called hemoglobin.

An A1C level of 7% or less means that your treatment plan is working and that your blood sugar was consistently within a healthy range. If your A1C level is higher than 7%, your blood sugar, on average, was above a healthy range. In this case, your health care provider may recommend a change in your diabetes treatment plan.

For some people, especially older adults and those with certain medical conditions, a higher A1C level of 8% or more may be appropriate.

How often you need the A1C test depends on the type of diabetes you have and how well you're managing your blood sugar. Most people with diabetes receive this test 2 to 4 times a year.

Treatment

Home treatment

Talk to your health care provider about managing your blood sugar. Understand how different treatments can help keep your glucose levels within your target range. Your health care provider may suggest the following:

1. Get physical. Regular exercise is often an effective way to control blood sugar. But don't exercise if you have ketones in your urine. This can drive your blood sugar even higher.
2. Take your medication as directed. If you develop hyperglycemia often, your health care provider may adjust the dosage or timing of your medication.
3. Follow your diabetes eating plan. It helps to eat smaller portions and avoid sugary beverages and frequent snacking. If you're having trouble sticking to your meal plan, ask your health care provider or dietitian for help.
4. Check your blood sugar. Monitor your blood glucose as directed by your health care provider. Check more often if you're sick or if you're concerned about severe hyperglycemia or hypoglycemia.
5. Adjust your insulin doses. Changes to your insulin program or a supplement of short-acting insulin can help control hyperglycemia. A supplement is an extra dose of insulin used to help temporarily correct a high blood sugar level. Ask your health care provider how often you need an insulin supplement if you have high blood sugar.

Emergency treatment for severe hyperglycemia

If you have signs and symptoms of diabetic ketoacidosis or hyperosmolar hyperglycemic state, you may be treated in the emergency room or admitted to the hospital. (4p4) Emergency treatment can lower your blood sugar to a normal range. Treatment usually includes:

Fluid replacement. You'll receive fluids — usually through a vein (intravenously) — until your body has the fluids it needs. This replaces fluids you've lost through urination. It also helps dilute the extra sugar in your blood.

Electrolyte replacement. Electrolytes are minerals in your blood that are necessary for your tissues to work properly.

A lack of insulin can lower the level of electrolytes in your blood. You'll receive electrolytes through your veins to help keep your heart, muscles and nerve cells working the way they should.

Insulin therapy. Insulin reverses the processes that cause ketones to build up in your blood. Along with fluids and electrolytes, you'll receive insulin therapy — usually through a vein.

Nutritional treatment in the critically-ill complicated patient

Hyperglycemia is a common complication of artificial nutrition due to the intravenous infusion of glucose and the metabolic stress associated with acute illness. The fat excess of obese subjects also contributes to insulin resistance, leading to hyperglycemia in a high proportion of these patients. The transcendence of hyperglycemia and plasma glucose variability is their relation to adverse clinical outcomes, including mortality. Blood glucose measuring is recommended when the patient enters the ICU or when artificial nutrition is started and a minimum of every 4 h during the first 2 days of admission. More frequent monitoring should be granted to unstable patients and, ideally, with arterial or venous samples. Capillary glycemic control is less reliable in the critical setting.

Although the exact range of blood glucose levels is not definitely established, there is a general consensus that the goal is keeping values between 140 and 180 mg/dL, and the upper desired level should not exceed 180 mg/dL. The main concern is avoiding hypoglycemia because although some trials offered promising results with lower blood glucose levels, especially in surgical patients (80–110 mg/dL) [37,38], these results were not confirmed in later publications. No diminished mortality could be demonstrated in the VISEP Trial despite the risk of severe hypoglycemia. In fact, in the large NICE-Sugar Trial, where more than 6000 patients were included with a blood glucose target of 80–100 mg/dL, a tight glucose control group had higher mortality at 90 days (27.5% vs. 24.9%; P = .02).

Treatment of choice for hyperglycemia in ICU is intravenous insulin, which must be adjusted to maintain blood glucose in the mentioned interval while reducing the risk of hypoglycemia. The amount of calories infused may influence insulin requirements, reducing both length (3.2 ± 2.7 vs. 8 ± 0.5 days) and dose (36.1 ± 47.1 UI vs. 61.1 ± 61 IU). A widely extended method for controlling hyperglycemia is starting intravenous insulin infusion at a minimum of 0.5 UI/h and then adjusting it in accordance with capillary glucose measurements every 1–2 h. An alternative could be to add insulin to parenteral nutrition, to provide both glucose and insulin simultaneously. When enteral nutrition is the chosen support, subcutaneous insulin is also acceptable, with NPH showing the best results. In our experience, subcutaneous regimens with once-daily basal insulin plus rapid-acting analogs every 4–6 h is a valid method for treating postsurgical patients.

There is no preference for specific diets for the nutritional support of diabetic patients, given the scarce evidence to prove a clinical benefit, although ESPEN remarks the possibility of improving glucose profiles and some economic advantage with enteral diabetes-specific preparations.

As your body returns to normal, your health care provider will consider what may have triggered the severe hyperglycemia. Depending on the circumstances, you may need additional tests and treatment.

14 Easy Ways to Lower Blood Sugar Levels Naturally

Exercising regularly, managing stress, and eating more foods high in fiber and probiotics may help lower blood sugar levels. However, these lifestyle adjustments do not replace medical treatment for diabetes or other metabolic conditions.

Your body usually manages your blood sugar levels by producing insulin, which allows your cells to use the circulating sugar in your blood. However, multiple factors can impair blood sugar management and lead to hyperglycemia (high blood sugar).

Blood sugar management is especially important for people with diabetes, as the condition may lead to limb and life threatening complications.

Here are 14 easy and evidence-backed ways to naturally lower blood sugar levels.

Exercise and movement throughout the day

Regular exercise and physical activity can help you manage your weight and increaseTrusted Source insulin sensitivity. Increased insulin sensitivity means your cells can use the glucose in your bloodstream more effectively.

Exercise also helps your muscles use blood sugar for energy and muscle contraction.

If you have problems with blood sugar management, consider routinely checking your levels before and after exercising. This will help you learn how your body responds to different activities and keep your blood sugar levels from getting too high or low.

You can still benefit from shorter sessions even if you have trouble dedicating more time to exercise throughout the week. For example, try aiming for 10-minute exercise sessions 3 times a day for 5 days, with the goal of 150 minutes per week.

So-called "exercise snacksTrusted Source" also help prevent the damage that sitting for prolonged periods can do. Exercise snacks mean you break up your sitting time every 30 minutes for just a few minutes throughout the day. Some recommended exercises include light walking or simple resistance exercises, like squats or leg raises.

Other useful forms of exercise include:

- weightlifting
- brisk walking
- running
- biking
- dancing
- hiking
- swimming
- jumping jacks
- half squats

Any activity that gets you up and moving — regardless of the intensity — beats a sedentary lifestyle.

Manage your carb intake

Your carb intake strongly influences your blood sugar levels. Your body breaks carbs down into sugars, mainly glucose. Then, insulin helps your body use and store it for energy.

This process fails when you eat too many carbs or have insulin-function problems, and blood glucose levels can rise.

That's why the American Diabetes Association recommends that people with diabetes manage their carb intake by counting carbs and being aware of how many they need for daily activities.

Carb counting can help you plan your meals appropriately, improving trusted Source blood sugar management.

A low carb diet helps reduce blood sugar levels and prevent trusted Source spikes.

It's important to note that low carb and no-carb diets are different.

When monitoring your blood sugar, you can eat (and need) some carbs. However, prioritizing carbs from whole grains and unprocessed sources provides greater nutritional value while helping decrease blood sugar levels.

Eat more fiber

Fiber slows carb digestion and sugar absorption, promoting a more gradual rise in blood sugar levels.

There are two types of fiber: insoluble and soluble.

While both are important, soluble fiber has been explicitly shown trusted Source to improve blood sugar management, while insoluble fiber hasn't been shown to have this effect.

A high fiber diet can improve your body's ability to regulate and minimize blood sugar levels. This could help you trusted Source better manage type 1 diabetes.

Foods high in fiber include:

- vegetables
- fruits
- legumes
- whole grains

The recommended daily intake of fiber trusted Source is about 25 grams for females and 35 grams for males. That's about 14 grams for every 1,000 calories.

Drink water

Drinking enough water could help you keep your blood sugar levels within healthy ranges. In addition to preventing dehydration, it helps your kidneys flush out excess sugar through urine.

One 2021 review trusted Source of observational studies found that people who drank more water had a lower risk of developing high blood sugar levels.

Drinking water regularly may rehydrate the blood, lower blood sugar levels, and reduce diabetes risk.

Keep in mind that water and other zero-calorie drinks are better for hydration. Avoiding sugar-sweetened options is ideal, as these can raise blood glucose, drive unwanted weight gain, and increase trusted Source diabetes risk.

Implement portion management

Managing how much you eat can help you regulate your calorie intake and maintain a moderate weight.

Consequently, weight management promotes trusted Source healthy blood sugar levels and has been shown to reduce the risk of developing type 2 diabetes.

Monitoring your serving sizes also helps prevent blood sugar spikes.

You may manage portion sizes by:

- eating slowly
- measuring and weighing your food
- using smaller plates
- avoiding all-you-can-eat restaurants or those that serve large portions
- reading food labels and checking the serving sizes of each item
- keeping a food journal
- using a food-tracking phone app
- Choose low glycemic foods

The glycemic index (GI) measures how quickly carbs break down during digestion and how rapidly your body absorbs them. This affects how quickly your blood sugar levels rise.

The GI divides foods into low, medium, and high GI scores and ranks them on a scale of 0 to 100. Low GI foods have a ranking of 55 or lower trusted Source. Consistently eating low GI foods may reduce blood sugar levels in people with diabetes.

Some examples of foods with a low to moderate GI include:

- bulgur
- barley
- unsweetened Greek yogurt
- oats
- beans
- lentils
- legumes
- whole wheat pasta
- non-starchy vegetables

Furthermore, adding protein or healthy fats to your plate helps minimize blood sugar spikes after a meal.

Focusing on the overall quality of the food is a better approach than eliminating or adding specific food groups.

Manage your stress levels

Stress can affect your blood sugar levels. When stressed, your body secretes hormones called glucagon and cortisol, which cause blood sugar levels to rise.

Stress management strategies may include:

- exercise
- meditation
- mindfulness
- deep breathing
- journaling
- arts and crafts
- psychotherapy
- your favorite hobbies

Exercises and relaxation methods, like yoga trusted Source and mindfulness-based stress reduction trusted Source, may also help correct insulin secretion problems among people with chronic diabetes receiving medical treatment.

Track your blood sugar levels

Monitoring blood glucose levels can help you better manage trusted Source them. You can do so at home using a portable blood glucose meter, known as a glucometer. You can discuss this option with a doctor.

Keeping track lets you determine whether to adjust your meals or medications. It also helps you learn how your body reacts to certain foods.

Try measuring your daily levels and keeping track of the numbers in a log. It may also be more helpful to track your blood sugar in pairs. For example, before and after exercise or before and 2 hours after a meal.

This can show you whether you need to make small changes to a meal if it spikes your blood sugar rather than avoiding your favorite meals altogether.

Some adjustments include swapping a starchy side for non-starchy veggies or limiting them to a handful.

Get enough quality sleep

Less than optimal sleeping habits and a lack of rest can affect trusted Source blood sugar levels and insulin sensitivity, increasing the chance of developing type 2 diabetes. They can also increase appetite and promote weight gain.

Sleep deprivation also raises trusted Source levels of cortisol, which plays an essential role in blood sugar management.

Adequate sleep is about both quantity and quality. Adults are advised to get 7 to 8 hours trusted Source of high quality sleep per night.

To improve the quality of your sleep, try to:

- follow a consistent sleep schedule
- avoid caffeine and alcohol before bed
- get physical activity throughout the day
- cut down on screen time before bed
- keep your bedroom cool and comfortable
- limit your naps during the day
- use soothing scents, such as lavender
- avoid working or studying in your bedroom if possible
- take a warm bath or shower before bed
- try meditation or guided imagery

Eat foods rich in chromium and magnesium

High blood sugar levels and diabetes have been linked trusted Source to micronutrient deficiencies, including chromium and magnesium.

Chromium is involved in carb and fat metabolism. It may enhance insulin's action, thus aiding blood sugar regulation.

Chromium-rich foods include:

- beef, chicken, and turkey
- whole grains, such as barley
- fruits and vegetables, like green beans and apples
- almonds

However, the mechanisms behind this proposed connection are not entirely known. More research is needed.

Magnesium also benefits blood sugar level regulation. Diets rich in magnesium are associated trusted Source with a significantly reduced risk of diabetes.

In contrast, low magnesium levels may lead to insulin resistance and decreased glucose tolerance in people with diabetes.

You likely won't benefit from magnesium supplements if you already eat plenty of magnesium-rich foods and have adequate blood magnesium levels.

Magnesium-rich foods include:

- dark leafy greens
- squash and pumpkin seeds
- tuna
- whole grains
- dark chocolate
- bananas
- avocados
- beans

Be careful with foods marketed as 'medicinal'

Multiple foods and plants are known to have medicinal properties. However, the quality of evidence on these ingredients is low due to insufficient human studies or small sample sizes. Therefore, no conclusive recommendations trusted Source can be made regarding their use.

Some of the foods touted to have anti-diabetes effects include:

Apple cider vinegar: According to a 2014 article trusted Source, this ingredient may reduce blood sugar levels by delaying the emptying of your stomach after a meal. A 2020 study trusted Source in rats also found that apple cider vinegar reduced blood sugar spikes. The authors concluded that the use of apple vinegar could help prevent metabolic disorders, like diabetes, in individuals eating a high calorie diet.

Cinnamon: This spice is said to improve trusted Source blood sugar levels by enhancing insulin sensitivity and slowing the breakdown of carbs in your digestive tract. This moderates the rise in blood sugar after a meal. Nevertheless, more research is needed.

Berberine: Research trusted Source suggests this compound lowers blood sugar by stimulating enzymes' breakdown of glucose, promoting your tissue's use of sugar and increasing insulin production. More studies are needed.

Fenugreek seeds: Like the other foods on this list, more high quality studies in humans are needed, but there is some evidence trusted Source that fenugreek may help support blood sugar management.

It's essential to talk with your doctor before adding any of these foods to your diet if you're already taking diabetes medications, as some herbal supplements may negatively interact with them.

Finally, the Food and Drug Administration (FDA) does not regulate supplements like it regulates prescription medications. Purchasing supplements that an independent lab has tested for purity and ingredient content is important.

Manage your weight

Maintaining your doctor's recommended weight range for your age and height promotes healthy blood sugar levels and reduces your risk of developing diabetes.

If you have overweight or obesity, research shows that even a 5%Trusted Source reduction in body weight can improve your blood sugar regulation and reduce the need for diabetes medication.

For example, if a person weighs 200 pounds (91 kilograms) and loses 10 to 14 pounds (4.5 to 6 kilograms), they may see significant improvements in their blood sugar levels.

What's more, losing more than 5% of your initial weight may benefit your HbA1c readings. These are used as indicators of your blood sugar levels over the past 3 months.

Eat healthy snacks more frequently

Spreading your meals and snacks throughout the day may help you avoid high and low blood sugar levels. Snacking between meals may also reduce trusted Source your risk of type 2 diabetes.

Smaller, more frequent meals throughout the day could improve trusted Source insulin sensitivity and lower blood sugar levels. In addition, eating smaller meals and healthy snacks throughout the day may lower HbA1c readings, indicating improvements in blood sugar levels over the previous 3 months.

Eat probiotic-rich foods

Probiotics are friendly bacteria with numerous health benefits, including improved blood sugar regulation. Probiotics may lower fasting blood sugar, HbA1c, and insulin resistance in people with type 2 diabetes.

Interestingly, a 2016 study found that improvements in blood sugar levels are more significant in people who consume multiple species of probiotics for at least 8 weeks.

Probiotic-rich foods include fermented foods, such as:

- yogurt, as long as the label states that it contains live active cultures
- kefir
- tempeh
- sauerkraut
- kimchi

Healthy Foods For Diabetes

Managing diabetes can reduce the risks for diabetes complications. Healthy eating is key. In this blog, we'll cover some healthy foods for diabetes.

The American Diabetes Association recommends a healthy meal plan for preventing/controlling diabetes. This plan is generally the same as healthy eating for anyone – low in saturated fat, moderate in salt and sugar, with meals based on lean protein, non-starchy vegetables, whole grains, healthy fats, and fruit.

The list of foods below provided by the American Diabetes Association is rich in vitamins, minerals, antioxidants and fiber that are good for overall health and may also help prevent disease. They're healthy foods for diabetes, plus they're all foods that AmpleHarvest.org helps supply to communities.

Dark Green Leafy Vegetables

Spinach, collards, and kale are dark green leafy vegetables packed with vitamins and minerals such as vitamins A, C, E, and K, iron, calcium and potassium. These powerhouse foods are low in calories and carbohydrates too. Try adding dark leafy vegetables to salads, soups and stews.

Citrus Fruit

Grapefruits, oranges, lemons and limes or pick your favorites to get part of your daily dose of fiber, vitamin C, folate and potassium.

Sweet Potatoes

A starchy vegetable packed full of vitamin A and fiber. They are also a good source of vitamin C and potassium.

Craving something sweet? Try a sweet potato in place of a regular potato and sprinkle cinnamon on top.

Berries

Which are your favorites: blueberries, strawberries or another variety? Regardless, they are all packed with antioxidants, vitamins and fiber. Berries can be a great option to satisfy your sweet tooth and they provide an added benefit of vitamin C, vitamin K, manganese, potassium and fiber.

Tomatoes

The good news is that no matter how you like your tomatoes, pureed, raw, or in a sauce, you're eating vital nutrients like vitamin C, vitamin E and potassium.

In many food insecure households, fresh food is difficult to come by. It is common for food pantries to distribute non-perishable items such as canned goods and boxed items for storage reasons. These products typically have a high-sodium and sugar content and lower nutritional value than fresh fruits and veggies.

DIET

The diet of a diabetic patient does not need to be restrictive. The diet should instead be healthy, rich in nutrients, low in fat, low in calories, and alkaline in nature. A diet that facilitates diabetes reversal is the best eating plan for anyone.

In the modern diet, many items are taking a toll on health. To name a few…

Refined sugar: It has been proven over several studies that refined sugar causes insulin resistance and fatty liver. It has also been proven to have close links to obesity, diabetes, and heart disease. So whether you have diabetes or not, if you want a healthy life, you should avoid refined sugar.

Refined grains: Some studies similar to the one by Dr. Barnard have proven that refined grain leads to rapid spikes in blood sugar, insulin resistance, and weight gain. It would be best if you avoided having refined grains as the first meal of your day.

Refined Oils: Refined oils are considered high in inflammatory Omega-6 fatty acids; these oils increase inflammation and oxidative damage. A healthy body decreases inflammation and reduces oxidative damage by avoiding refined oils.

Trans Fats: The last but not least on the list is trans fat. Trans fat is extremely harmful; artificial fats are found in processed foods and are linked to many serious diseases, especially heart disease. Trans fat also contributes to diabetes. By eliminating processed food and trans fat in your body, you will achieve better insulin sensitivity.

A low-fat plant-based diet, also known as Vegan Diet, profoundly impacts metabolic conditions like Diabetes. Clinical researchers like Barnard, associate professor of medicine at the George Washington University School of Medicine and Health Sciences, and Dr. Joel Fuhrman, Director of Research at the Nutritional Research Foundation, have studied vegan diet for decades.

And based on the studies they've conducted over the past few decades, there is conclusive proof that a vegan diet is three times more effective in controlling our blood sugar than other diets usually recommended for people with diabetes by doctors.

For those new to the vegan diet, it is a vegetarian diet that excludes animal products like meat, eggs, dairy, and other animal-derived ingredients. To understand why a vegan diet is so crucial in reversing diabetes, we first need to understand the cause of diabetes and what effect animal products have on our bodies.

We all know diabetes is a type of malfunction when our body cannot use the sugar formed due to digestion. Our blood sugar levels are dependent on the production of the hormone insulin from the pancreas. People who have type 2 diabetes are insulin resistant. Insulin helps in transporting glucose. The hormone binds to a receptor on the cell wall, opening a passage that allows glucose to enter the cell. The cell then metabolizes this glucose to use it as fuel to perform its various tasks.

Dietary causes of diabetes are :

(1) Fat interfering with hormones,

(2) Acidic and inflamed system and

(3) Lack of micronutrients [vitamins, minerals, phytonutrients, antioxidants, nutraceuticals, etc.

If you can fix your diet to remove these three irritants, you will see significant improvement in your blood sugar levels. Based on clinical studies by Dr. Neal Barnard, by adopting a low-fat vegetarian diet free of all animal products and added vegetable oils, individuals can lower their cholesterol, reduce their blood pressure, lose weight and attain better control over blood sugar. The reason is simple. A low-fat vegetarian diet (vegan diet without added vegetable oils) reduces the fat interfering with your hormones which will allow insulin that you naturally produce to bind correctly to the cell wall opening passage to allow for glucose to enter the cell. A vegan diet is also naturally abundant in vitamins, minerals, and phytonutrients. Now, if you focus on specific vegetables, you can also reduce the acidity in your body, reducing the inflammation in your system while providing antioxidants and nutraceuticals.

We typically start the day with a cup of tea or coffee in the morning. Usually, that is the first thing we consume on an empty stomach. Unfortunately, everyone, including healthy individuals, builds up acidity overnight. Both tea and coffee are acidic, so we increase our acidity by consuming tea or coffee first thing in the morning. Instead, the first thing you should do to start your day is to reduce the acidity buildup overnight with a nutrient-dense green smoothie that will help alkalize your body. A recipe for this stunningly nutrient-dense alkalizing green smoothie can be found here.

EXERCISES

Yoga & Anti-Gravity Exercises for Managing Blood Sugar

Yoga exercises are a great way to manage blood sugar levels for diabetic patients. They help to improve flexibility, reduce stress, and increase overall strength and balance. Additionally, yoga can help to improve blood circulation and reduce inflammation throughout the body. Anti-gravity exercises, such as aerial or inversion yoga, are also beneficial for managing blood sugar levels. These exercises help to improve circulation and reduce stress, while also strengthening the muscles and improving balance. Both yoga and anti-gravity exercises are excellent tools for managing blood sugar levels in diabetic patients.

Exercises help our bodies utilize the insulin hence helping diabetic control their blood sugars better. There are many benefits of exercising ranging from healthy heart, strong bones, stress reducer, lowers blood pressure, improves cholesterol, improves blood circulation to controlling your blood sugar levels.

Anti-gravity exercises

Anti-gravity resistance exercises can be performed in the comfort of your home or a hotel room when traveling. You do not need a gym or fancy equipment to perform these exercises.

Yoga exercises

It is well known that regular yoga practice can help reduce stress levels, enhance mobility, lower blood pressure and improve overall well-being. It is these benefits that many health experts believe can improve diabetes management and protect against other related medical conditions such as heart disease. Here you will find easy-to-follow instructional videos to help reduce your blood sugar with yoga exercises.

MEDITATION

Meditation and Its Benefits for Diabetes Management

Meditation is a powerful tool for managing blood sugar levels in diabetic patients. It helps to reduce stress and improve overall wellbeing, while also improving blood circulation and reducing inflammation throughout the body. Additionally, meditation can help to improve mental clarity and focus, and promote a sense of calm and relaxation. By incorporating meditation into their daily routine, diabetic patients can better manage their blood sugar levels and lead a healthier lifestyle.

Meditation is training the mind to attain consciousness and to concentrate on the awareness around it. Meditation is immensely helpful for reversing diabetes by relieving stress which is one of the contributing factors for diabetes. By lowering stress, you will attain better control of your blood glucose levels.

Benefits of meditation, to name a few:

- It encourages a healthy lifestyle.
- It increases happiness.
- It slows aging.
- It improves cardiovascular and immune health.
- Types of meditation, to name a few –
- Mindful meditation
- Dynamic meditation
- Sahaj meditation
- Guided meditation

Any meditation you practice regularly is good for you. It depends on your preference. It would be best if you meditate regularly.

Dynamic meditation is considered favorable for diabetic patients as it is easy to follow and also provides physical exercise while meditating. Reduced stress, better diabetes control, lower blood pressure, lower blood glucose levels, greater self-awareness, better relationships, improved focus in other areas of your life, and less depression and anxiety are all potential benefits of including meditation in your routine. You will find easy-to-follow instructional videos to help reduce your blood sugar with meditation.

Conclusion

Diabetes is a slow killer with no known curable treatments. However, its complications can be reduced through proper awareness and timely treatment. Three major complications are related to blindness, kidney damage and heart attack. It is important to keep the blood glucose levels of patients under strict control for avoiding the complications. One of the difficulties with tight control of glucose levels in the blood is that such attempts may lead to hypoglycemia that creates much severe complications than an increased level of blood glucose. Researchers now look for alternative methods for diabetes treatment. The goal of this paper is to give a general idea of the current status of diabetes research. The author believes that diabetes is one of the highly demanding research topics of the new century and wants to encourage new researchers to take up the challenges. Hyperglycemia is the underlying cause of diabetes and causes a progressive decline of β-cell function leading to β-cell exhaustion and eventually β-cell demise and dysfunction. Also, it is involved in the generation of free radicals and the depletion of the antioxidant system, which result in oxidative stress. Oxidative stress has been implicated in the etiology of diabetes complications, therefore, the abatement of hyperglycemia and annihilation of oxidative stress provide an auspicious alternative in the treatment of diabetes and its complications. Dacryodes edulis possesses phytochemicals that have the potential to act as antihyperglycemic and antioxidative agents, thus, protecting against β-cell exhaustion and dysfunction. Various mechanisms have been proposed for the protective ability of D. edulis in diabetes pathology, which range from delaying carbohydrate digestion and absorption and β-cell regeneration to increasing insulin secretion, increasing glucose uptake and utilization, regulating lipid metabolism, scavenging free radicals, and increasing the antioxidant defense system. Various studies have attributed these potentials to its phytochemistry, particularly polyphenols. Therefore D. edulis may be employed as a potent functional food and/or nutraceutical in the treatment and management of diabetes and its complications.